Clean

Jumpstart Weight Loss with 70 Clean Eating Recipes

The Healthy Cookbook for the Busy Professional

Daisy Williams

This book is dedicated to anyone who is struggling with weight or health issues. Clean recipes that you enjoy will keep you focused on eating healthy.

TABLE OF CONTENTS

PUBLISHER'S NOTES

Disclaimer

This publication is intended to provide helpful and informative material. It is not intended to diagnose, treat, cure, or prevent any health problem or condition, nor is intended to replace the advice of a physician. No action should be taken solely on the contents of this book. Always consult your physician or qualified health-care professional on any matters regarding your health and before adopting any suggestions in this book or drawing inferences from it.

The author and publisher specifically disclaim all responsibility for any liability, loss or risk, personal or otherwise, which is incurred as a consequence, directly or indirectly, from the use or application of any contents of this book.

Any and all product names referenced within this book are the trademarks of their respective owners. None of these owners have sponsored, authorized, endorsed, or approved this book.

Always read all information provided by the manufacturers' product labels before using their products. The author and publisher are not responsible for claims made by manufacturers.

Print Edition 2014

CHAPTER 1: WHAT IS CLEAN EATING?

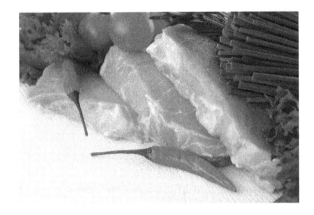

Everyone seems to currently be interested in clean eating. Diet fads come and go but clean eating is a lifestyle change. Diets tend to focus on restricting food intake and short term weight loss but clean eating is about long term health. The simple truth is that you cannot become healthy if you don't eat healthy.

The right foods are the ticket to better health. If you eat a lot of processed foods loaded with sugar and fats, your body is going to show it. If you eat healthy, whole, fresh foods, your skin, soul and body will glow of good health and give you ongoing energy.

There are three methods for clean eating.

Method 1 – Eat regular meals when hungry or only when necessary.

Many people are simply looking to get rid of the chemicals from their diets and bodies and turn to eating clean. They focus on overall health and not losing weight. They avoid any type of food that is processed and eat regular meals.

Method 2 – Eat about six small meals a day.

Eat food that comes directly from nature. Eat foods that come off trees, bushes, vines or plants. The concept involves staying away from any food that humans have altered in any way at all.

Include meats that are straight from the butcher and are whole meats. Don't use meat products that are pre-packaged because you have no idea what is in them. If possible, buy your meats whole and grind them at home. You might be surprised to find out what's really in ground turkey meat. The other option is to buy turkey breasts and have your butcher grind them for you. Most are more than willing to accommodate regular customers.

Enjoy plenty of grains. Eat the ones that are complete and not broken down. Stick with whole wheat, whole grains and brown rice.

Read all food labels. You might think you are eating good breads because you pick up the package and it says "whole grain". But, take a look at the ingredients. If you see white flour down second or third on the list, it's not the best bread to choose.

Eat foods with fewer ingredients. Try to buy foods that have less than six ingredients on the ingredients list. Make sure you know what all the ingredients are. If you find "mystery ingredients" like "spices", call the company and ask them what their spices consist of. If it includes anything other than spices and herbs, avoid it. Additionally, if you cannot pronounce an ingredient, you probably shouldn't eat it.

Eating six small meals a day may seem like a lot when you start, but you are also consuming smaller portions. To increase your success rate as a beginner, plan and prepare your food for the day and schedule when you are going to eat.

Method 3 – Eat three regular meals and one snack during the day for a total of four meals. With this method, you eat every four hours.

Clean eating might seem overwhelming to begin with, especially if you have a lot of changes to make with your current eating habits. Take baby steps. Making small changes each day is the best way to transition to a healthier eating regimen. Don't get upset with yourself if you make mistakes along the way because everyone does.

Some people are so accustomed to processed foods that they have a tough time with the natural flavor of real food. These people usually claim that they don't like the taste of vegetables or anything that is healthy. If this is you, listen up. Your taste buds will definitely change if you stick with eating clean. Over time you will find that the processed, unhealthy foods and sweets that you use to crave don't taste as good as you remember them to.

So, are you excited about clean eating and wondering how to start? Below are some steps that will help with a smooth transition to leave those old eating habits in the past and start clean eating.

Start off by stocking a clean eating pantry. Add plenty of fruits and vegetables. Add some lean meat such as fish and chicken breast. Consider adding some frozen vegetables and fruits as well. Check the ingredients to make sure the frozen foods have no added sugar. It's a good idea to stock the refrigerator and freezer with clean foods so you are not running to the store constantly for fresh foods. Consider making some things ahead of time, such as a whole wheat pie crust, so you can put a clean eating quiche together quickly when you're busy. Clean eating pizza dough, casseroles and other dishes can be made ahead of time as well. Preparation is the key to clean eating.

Clean out all the food in your refrigerator and cabinets. Read all the ingredients, and throw out anything that has ingredients that need to go. Be ruthless. Make sure you only keep foods that have ingredients you recognize and no more than six ingredients in them.

Next, make your grocery list and stock up on all your new clean eating foods. While shopping, think about the value of preparation time when it comes to clean eating. It's a lot easier to stick to the plan when you have your chopped vegetables and fruit ready to grab out of the refrigerator. Marinate some chicken breasts in zip lock bags, and freeze them so you can pull them out as you need them. Set some time aside to prepare your foods ahead of time for the week.

Give yourself some time to adjust to clean eating. Keep in mind that even though it's a big change for anyone, almost all recipes can be changed to a clean eating lifestyle. Even your favorite foods like pizza, ice cream, cakes and cookies can be made with clean eating ingredients. If you go into clean eating with a good attitude, you will do great!

CHAPTER 2: THE BENEFITS OF EATING CLEAN

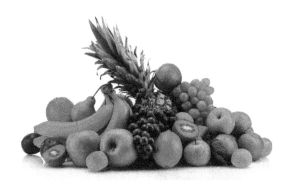

Clean eating involves eliminating processed food from your diet. Instead of focusing on weight loss goals, eating clean is more about becoming healthy. A clean diet can remove the toxins from your body and help you feel better. To eat clean, your diet should consist of fruits, vegetables, whole grains, low-fat dairy products and meat from free-range animals. You can benefit from eating clean in a number of ways.

More Energy

Eating healthy food can make you feel better. Adding vegetables, fruits and lean protein to your diet can balance your energy levels, which will leave you feeling great. Your body will start absorbing nutrients more efficiently, and you will feel more energetic. Since healthy foods promote cell growth, your skin, hair and nails will also become healthier.

Easier to Maintain a Healthy Weight

Eating whole foods instead of processed foods is the best way to maintain a healthy weight. Even if you spend hours in the gym, you must still eat a diet that is rich in vegetables, fruits, whole grains and lean meat to maintain a healthy figure. It only takes a few weeks of eating clean for you to start noticing a positive change within your body. Consuming less sodium and sugar makes it easier for you to control your weight. Besides that, you will also discover that exercising is easier once you reach a healthy weight.

A Stronger Immune System

Nutritious foods are full of vitamins, minerals and antioxidants; therefore, you can build a stronger immune system by adopting a clean diet. Having a good immune system is the best way to fight off illnesses before they even start. When you do get sick, having a good immune system will help you recover quickly. The best way to ensure that your immune system is running at an optimal level is to drink 8 to 10 glasses of water per day and to eat lots of fruits and vegetables.

Better Mental Awareness

Studies have shown that junk food clouds the mind and causes people to feel sluggish. Eating healthy is the best way to prevent this from happening. In fact eating products that are high in omega-3 fatty acids will help keep the brain functioning at top capacity. Switching to a clean diet can even lower your risk of diabetes and heart disease. Healthy foods encourage good blood flow to the brain, which is why a clean diet leads to better mental awareness.

Your brain needs the right amount of nutrients to function properly. Besides protein, you even need to consume healthy fats and sugar. Start eating more fruits and dark-skinned vegetables to protect your brain cells. Kale, broccoli, spinach and eggplants are great vegetables to eat because they are full of antioxidants. Some of the best fruits to consume include strawberries, blueberries, grapes and blackberries. You should also add cold-water fish to your diet for the omega-3 fatty acids. Nuts are also good for the brain because they have high levels of vitamin E.

Sleep More Peacefully

Healthy foods calm the nervous system, which triggers a sleep-inducing hormonal response. Therefore, adopting a clean diet will help you achieve a deeper sleep at night. Scientific research has shown that obesity rates and sleep deprivation share a connection. You should strive to get between seven and nine hours of sleep per night so that your body can function properly. Getting the proper amount of sleep helps your body build and repair muscle, which is essential if you exercise routinely. In addition, good sleeping patterns will sharpen your focus and help your body establish muscle memory.

Less Trans-Fat in Your Diet

Most doctors think that trans-fat is the worst type of fat for the body. Nearly 80 percent of trans-fat comes from processed foods, so eating a clean diet is the best way to avoid consuming too much of it. Trans-fat can increase the bad cholesterol levels in your body, which can cause you to develop cardiovascular-related health issues. Besides eating more fruits and vegetables, make sure to cut down on the amount of salt and sugar that you add to your food. According to scientists, reducing your dietary salt intake can help you prevent hypertension or death from heart disease.

Feel Full for Longer

Whole foods can keep you satisfied longer than processed food. In fact, you are less likely to pig out on junk food when you eat a clean diet. Being able to avoid the junk food temptation will make your life easier. Many unhealthy products such as cookies or candy can actually make you feel hungrier. Although it may take a few weeks, your body will eventually become used to eating a clean diet. Overtime, your body will start to crave healthy food instead of unhealthy food. For example, you may start to crave an apple instead of a bag of chips.

Since clean eating has numerous benefits, you should take action and implement clean eating and a healthier lifestyle today. It will only take a few short weeks for you to notice a significant improvement in the way your body looks and feels. Rather than thinking of clean eating as a diet, you should think of it as a lifestyle change. Change is hard so don't try to change your eating habits overnight. Start by making small changes. For example, start by incorporating more fruits and vegetables into your daily life.

CHAPTER 3: 10 FILLING CLEAN EATING BREAKFAST RECIPES

Though many people ignore the saying "breakfast is the most important meal of the day", eating a healthy meal in the morning is tremendously important to optimum health and nutrition. Clean eating is a method many people are turning to in our world full of processed foods, but breakfast can be tricky. Newcomers to clean eating are more than likely used to chemically-laden breakfast cereals or quick workout drinks. While these foods have their benefits, they lower the health of your body. Here are ten clean eating breakfast recipes that will fill you up until lunch.

SIMPLE OATMEAL

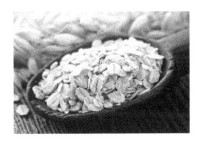

Ingredients:
½ cup pecans or walnuts
Small splash of pure vanilla extract
1/3 cup honey
2 tsp. cinnamon
½ cup plain rolled oats
⅔ cup organic milk

Directions:

1. Heat the milk on high (stovetop).
2. Upon boiling, drop in the oats and turn down the heat, letting the mixture simmer for two minutes.
3. Add the remaining ingredients and serve.

BLUEBERRY BAKED OATMEAL

Ingredients:

1½ cups blueberries

2 tsp. pure vanilla extract

3 tbsp. butter (melted)

1 large egg

2 cups organic milk

1 tsp. cinnamon

½ cup chopped pecans

1 tsp. baking powder

½ cup maple syrup (pure)

2 cups rolled oats

½ tsp. sea salt

Directions:

1. Preheat the oven to 375 degrees and use nonstick cooking spray to coat a glass baking dish.
2. In a bowl, combine the dry ingredients.
3. In a separate bowl, combine the wet ingredients.
4. Pour half the blueberries on the bottom of the baking dish, covering with the dry ingredients.
5. Top with the wet mixture and the remaining berries.
6. Let cook for 40 minutes, or until the top is a light golden brown.

OATMEAL HONEY MUFFINS

Ingredients:
¾ cup(s) rolled oats
¾ cup(s) whole-wheat flour
¾ cup(s) all-purpose flour
2 tsp. baking powder
½ tsp. sea salt
½ tsp. ground cinnamon
¼ tsp. baking soda
2 eggs
1/3 cup(s) organic honey
1/2 cup milk of choice
¼ cup vegetable oil

Directions:
1. Combine and mix oats, flours, baking powder, salt, cinnamon and soda.
2. Beat eggs, honey, milk and oil together and mix well.
3. Pour honey mixture over dry ingredients.
4. Mix until moistened and spoon into oiled or non-stick muffin tins.
5. Bake at 375 degrees for 20 to 30 minutes.

BASIC GREEN SMOOTHIE

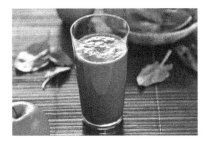

Ingredients:
1 cup of your favorite frozen fruit
1 apple, peeled and chopped

1 cup plain organic Greek yogurt

2 cups fresh greens (baby spinach is best for beginners)

Directions:

1. Throw all the ingredients into a high performance blender, like the Ninja or Vitamix.
2. Blend on high until your drink reaches a nice, smooth consistency that you are happy with.
3. Pour into large glass and enjoy!

PEANUT BUTTER BANANA SMOOTHIE

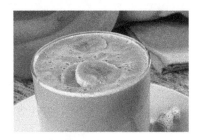

Ingredients:

½ cup ice cubes

¼ cup peanut butter

½ cup organic milk

½ banana

Directions:

1. Place all ingredients in a high-powered blender and mix until smooth and creamy.
2. Pour into a tall glass, kick back, relax, and enjoy the simple pleasure of a good breakfast.

BANANA WALNUT OATMEAL

Ingredients:

½ banana, mashed

¼ cup oats

½ cup organic milk

½ tbsp. crushed walnuts

Directions:
1. Combine banana, oats and milk in a microwavable bowl.
2. Microwave for about 3 minutes.
3. Stop to stir after each minute.
4. Add walnuts.

WHOLE-WHEAT ZUCCHINI MUFFINS

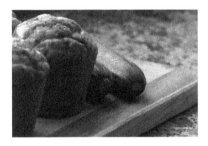

Ingredients:
3 cups grated zucchini

1 tsp. vanilla

½ cup honey

¾ cup olive oil

3 eggs

½ tsp. salt

¼ tsp. baking powder

1½ tsp. baking soda

1 tbsp. cinnamon

3 cups whole-wheat flour

Directions:
1. Preheat the oven to 325 degrees and grease your muffin pan thoroughly.
2. Blend your dry ingredients in a large bowl, being careful not to over mix.
3. Pour in all the wet ingredients (you'll only have the zucchini left to use).

4. Fold in the zucchini last; be sure it is well mixed with the rest of the ingredients.
5. Pour the batter into the muffin pan, filling about 3/4 full.
6. Bake for approximately 15 minutes.

Use a toothpick to check the middle of the muffin. It should be clean when pulled out.

WHOLE WHEAT TOAST & COTTAGE CHEESE

Ingredients:
2 slices whole-wheat bread
½ cup low fat cottage cheese

Directions:
1. Toast bread to desired level and top with cottage cheese.

OATMEAL PANCAKES
(That taste like French toast!)

Ingredients:
6 large egg whites
1 cup rolled oats, dry
1 cup low fat cottage cheese
2 tsp. sugar or sugar substitute (Xylitol or Crystalline)
1 tsp. vanilla

Directions:
1. In a blender or food processor, combine all the ingredients until the batter is smooth.
2. Heat a large non-stick griddle or frying pan over medium-low heat.
3. For each pancake pour about 1/4 cup of batter onto the griddle.
4. Flip pancakes twice when they start to get bubbly. Continue cooking until they are golden brown.
5. Repeat with remaining batter until gone.

6. Sprinkle additional cinnamon on top as desired.

*Makes 9 pancakes

WHOLE-WHEAT BANANA PANCAKES

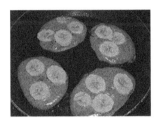

Ingredients:
2 stiffly beaten egg whites
2 egg yolks
2 ripe mashed bananas (have extra to slice and serve with pancakes)
1/3 cup canola oil
1½ cups milk
½ tsp. salt
¼ tsp. cinnamon
2 tsp. baking powder
2 cups whole wheat flour

Directions:
1. Preheat the griddle to three hundred and fifty degrees Fahrenheit.
2. In a big bowl whisk salt, cinnamon, baking powder and flour.
3. In another bowl combine egg yolks, bananas, oil and milk.
4. When done add it to the dry ingredients and combine. Fold the egg whites in gently.
5. Use some nonstick cooking spray to coat the griddle, then place approximately a third of the mix on the griddle until all the pancakes are on (space permitting).
6. Cook until the pancakes start to turn golden and bubbles are on the top (approximately two minutes).

7. Turn the pancakes over and let cook for another minute. Do this until all the pancakes are done.

CHAPTER 4: 10 GREAT CLEAN EATING LUNCH RECIPES

TUNA AND LETTUCE WRAPS

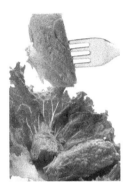

Ingredients:
6 ounces sushi-grade tuna
¼ cup nonfat plain yogurt
2 diced Roma tomatoes
8 small hearts of romaine
Sriracha hot chili sauce to taste

Directions:
1. Season tuna with salt and pepper to taste.
2. Heat a skillet over medium-high heat.
3. Sear tuna for 30 seconds per side, set aside to cool. Slice into eight pieces.
4. Whisk together Sriracha sauce and yogurt.
5. Place one piece of lettuce on a plate.
6. Place 2 tbsp tomatoes, top with 1 tsp. of Sriracha-yogurt mixture, and add one slice of tuna.
7. Roll lettuce gently, secure with a toothpick, and serve.

ITALIAN-GRILLED CHEESE

Ingredients:

2 slices whole-grain bread

2 tsp. pesto, prepared

1 ounce part-skim mozzarella cheese, sliced

1 plum tomato, sliced to desired thickness

2 large basil leaves

Directions:

1. Spread pesto on one side of each slice of bread.
2. Take one slice, pesto-side up, and layer cheese, basil, and tomato.
3. Top with first slice of bread, pesto-side down.
4. Grill in a Panini press.
5. Alternatively, spray a skillet with non-stick cooking spray, and cook sandwich on the stove.

CHICKEN AND STRAWBERRY PITA POCKET

Ingredients:

1 whole wheat pita pocket

3 oz. boneless chicken breast sliced

1 tbsp. olive oil

1 tbsp. reduced fat mayonnaise

½ cup shredded lettuce

4 fresh strawberries cleaned and slice

Directions:

1. Combine the chicken, olive oil, mayonnaise, lettuce and strawberries in a bowl and mix thoroughly.
2. Fill mixed ingredients in pita pockets and enjoy.

PROTEIN POWER SHAKE

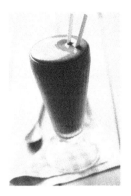

Ingredients:

8 ounces unsweetened soy milk

¼ cup chocolate protein powder

2 tbsp. ground flaxseeds

2 tbsp. cacao powder

1½ tbsp. fresh mint leaves

5 ice cubes

Directions:

1. Combine all ingredients in a blender.
2. Blend on high for one to two minutes.
3. Pour into a glass and enjoy.

TOMATO AND AVOCADO SANDWICH

Ingredientes:

Tomato

Avocado

Whole wheat bread

Directions:

1. Slice up tomato and avocado
2. Toast whole wheat bread
3. Combine ingredients and enjoy!

WHOLE GRAIN PASTA WITH CHICKEN

Ingredients:

2 chicken breast, cooked and chopped or sliced

1 cup cherry tomatoes, halved

½ cucumber, chopped

1 red bell pepper, chopped

4 oz. artichoke hearts

Mix the above ingredients together

Dressing Ingredients:

1 shallot, minced

1 7-oz container Greek yogurt

2 tbsp. reserved marinade from artichoke hearts

Directions:

1. Mix the dressing and put pour over the chicken.
2. Refrigerate and enjoy!

INSTANT TURKEY WRAP

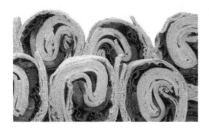

Ingredients:

Lettuce of your choice

Whole-wheat tortilla

Sliced turkey breast

Light sour cream

Tomato, sliced

Red onion, sliced (optional)

Peppers (optional)

Directions:

1. Evenly place the lettuce on the tortilla.
2. Overlap the turkey breast on top of the lettuce.
3. Spread one tbsp. of sour cream over the turkey.
4. Add tomatoes, onions and peppers/
5. Roll up the tortilla into a tight cylinder tucking in the sides.
6. Slice the wrap in half and enjoy!

CLEAN TACO

Ingredients:

1½ pounds lean ground turkey meat
2 tsp. garlic powder
2 tsp. chili powder
2 tsp.paprika
Pepper to taste

Optional Ingredients:

Avocado sliced
Lettuce, shredded
Black beans–no sugar added
Tomatoes–sliced
Onions–sliced
Olives–sliced
Low fat shredded cheese

Directions:

1. In a pan over medium heat cook turkey, garlic, chili, paprika, salt, and pepper until turkey is no longer pink and heated through.
2. In a bowl layer the turkey meat and any of the optional toppings.

TOMATO AND CHICKEN SANDWICH

Ingredients:
Grilled chicken breast
1 large beefsteak tomato
Lettuce
Red onion, thinly sliced
1 slice Swiss cheese

Directions:
1. Marinate chicken in light or fat free Italian dressing.
2. Slice chicken into one inch strips.
3. Place chicken between two thick slices of beefsteak tomato for a chicken sandwich that is light, full of protein and healthy.
4. Lettuce and thinly sliced red onion can also be added on top of the chicken and even a thin slice of Swiss cheese can be used to make this knife and fork sandwich even tastier.

ROASTED CHICKEN BREAST AND ASPARAGUS

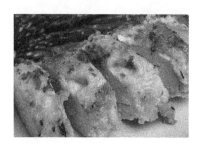

Ingredients:
Cooking spray
2 tbsp. Olive Oil
Asparagus, trimmed and cut into 1 inch pieces
¾ cups fresh basil chopped
3 Boneless, skinless chicken breasts cut into 2 inch cubes
½ cups chopped Roma tomatoes
8 Cloves of garlic thinly sliced
1 tbsp. freshly chopped Rosemary

Ground Pepper to taste

Directions:

1. Preheat oven to 400 degrees and spray large baking dish with cooking spray.
2. Add chicken, garlic, asparagus, tomatoes and olive oil.
3. Sprinkle top with Rosemary and garlic.
4. Bake for 20-30 minutes, turning occasionally until tender.

*Serves 3 to 4

CHAPTER 5: 10 QUICK TO PREPARE CLEAN EATING SNACK RECIPES

When hunger strikes, clean eating can pose a challenge for those who are unprepared to create fast, nutritious snacks without the unnecessary additives included in processed foods. Fortunately, many of the most delicious snacks can be prepared in a matter of minutes while using only natural and nutritious ingredients. Here are 10 clean eating snack recipes that are simple to prepare so anyone can maintain their clean eating style without sacrificing on time.

TRAIL MIX

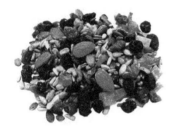

Known for its easy portability and ability to be modified, trail mix is a popular snack that can be taken to work or included in a lunchbox. When preparing this snack, be sure to modify it according to personal tastes. However, this recipe is sure to be a hit.

Ingredients:
1/8 cup dried fruit (assorted works well)
1/8 cup walnuts
2 tbsp. sunflower seeds

Sprinkle of dark chocolate chips or carobs

Directions:
1. Place all ingredients in a bowl and mix together.
2. Then, place into individual serving bags or eat immediately.

BANANA WRAP

For hungry children or adults who need a quick burst of energy, this snack can be prepared in a flash with clean ingredients most people have already on hand.

Ingredients:
1 banana
3 tbsp. peanut butter
1 whole wheat tortilla
Cinnamon to taste

Directions:
1. Spread the desired type of peanut butter on one tortilla.
2. Then, add a light sprinkle of cinnamon.
3. Place the banana in the middle of the tortilla and roll it up.

YOGURT PARFAIT

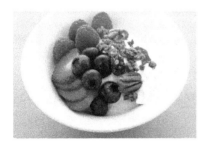

Although this recipe is often enjoyed as a dessert, it can also be served as a snack that is packed full of calcium and antioxidants.

Ingredients:
1 cup plain Greek yogurt

3 sliced strawberries
1/8 cup blueberries
1/8 cup raspberries
2 tbsp. granola

Directions:
1. Place ¼ cup of yogurt in a dish.
2. Then, create layers by alternating the addition of yogurt and assorted fruits.
3. Finish by topping the parfait with granola before serving.

PARMESAN-CRUSTED COLLARD CHIPS

Finding a replacement for a potato chip craving is not hard with this clean eating recipe. With only a few simple ingredients, even the strongest craving can be satisfied with the crunch of a collard green.

Ingredients:
1 head collard greens
1 tsp. lemon juice
1/8 cup grated Parmesan cheese
3 tbsp. olive oil
½ tsp. cayenne pepper
½ tsp. sea salt

Directions:
1. Begin by preheating the oven to 350 degrees.
2. Prep the collard greens by removing the stems and cutting leaves into 3-inch pieces.
3. In a large bowl, toss the greens with the olive oil, Parmesan cheese and lemon juice.
4. Once the greens are coated, season them with the cayenne pepper and sea salt.
5. Place the coated collard greens in a single layer on parchment paper-lined baking sheets.

6. Then bake for approximately 18 minutes or until they are crisp.

RAW BROCCOLI & RANCH DIP

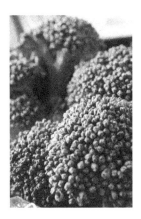

Ingredients:

2 cups raw broccoli

2 tbsp. low-fat ranch of your choice

Directions:

1. Wash broccoli thoroughly.
2. Dip in ranch and enjoy!

COTTAGE CHEESE, CINNAMON AND WALNUTS

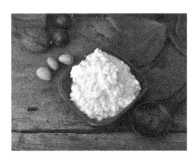

Ingredients:

1 cup low-fat cottage cheese

1 tbsp. chopped walnuts

¼ tsp. ground cinnamon

Directions:

1. Combine cottage cheese, walnuts and cinnamon.
2. Mix thoroughly and enjoy!

HEALTHY BANANA BERRY SMOOTHIE

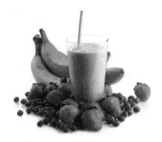

Ingredients:

1 cup frozen unsweetened mixed berries

1 cup non-fat milk

¼ cup fat free plain or vanilla yogurt

1 ripe banana

2 tbsp. flax seed

2 tbsp. vanilla whey protein powder

5-6 ice cubes

Directions:

1. Blend all ingredients until combined and serve.

STRING CHEESE & GRAPES

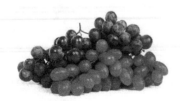

Ingredients:

1 cup of green or red seedless grapes

1 organic or light serving of string cheese

Directions:
1. Wash and dry grapes.
2. Peel and eat cheese

*This is an easy snack to take on the go for the kid in all of us.

GREEK YOGURT WITH CINNAMON

Ingredients:
6 ounces nonfat Greek yogurt

1 tsp. ground cinnamon

Directions:
1. Combine yogurt and cinnamon in a bowl.

FRESH VEGGIES AND DIP

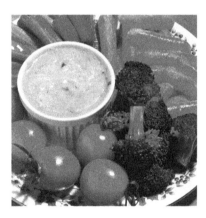

Ingredients:
1½ cups low-fat, plain Greek yogurt

1/3 cup crumbled feta cheese

2 tbsp. fresh lemon juice

2 tbsp. fresh dill, chopped

1 small clove garlic, minced

Kosher sea salt and pepper to taste

Fresh vegetables, chopped

Directions:

1. Combine all of the ingredients, minus the veggies, in a bowl.
2. Stir until ingredients are well blended.
3. Scoop dip into small serving dish and chill.
4. Enjoy dip with your favorite vegetables.

Chapter 6: 10 Light Clean Eating Salads

CHICKEN SALAD WITH GREEK YOGURT, DICED CELERY, AND WALNUTS

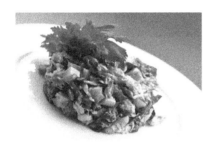

Ingredients:
2 chicken breasts, cooked and chopped

1½ cups Greek yogurt

1 stalk celery, diced

¼ cup walnuts

Sea salt and cracked black pepper to taste

Chopped spring onion for garnishing

Directions:
1. Combine the chicken, celery, and walnuts in a bowl.
1. Add the Greek yogurt and mix thoroughly.
2. Top with the chopped spring onion.
3. It can be eaten on its own, in a sandwich or pita.

COBB SALAD

Ingredients:
6 cups of chopped romaine heart lettuce

2 seeded and peeled ripe avocados, sliced into 1" pieces

1 skinless chicken breast, cooked and cubed

2 chopped vine-ripe tomatoes

2 peeled and sliced hard-boiled eggs

Cooking spray

2 cups of watercress with thick stems removed

2 ounces of blue cheese

¼ pound smoked ham

Dressing Ingredients:

½ cup olive oil

½ cup red-wine vinegar

1 tsp. of pure maple syrup or honey

Sea salt or kosher to taste

1/8 of black pepper

1 tsp. of lemon juice

1 tsp. of Dijon Mustard

1 small and minced clove garlic

Directions:

1. Combine all the dressing ingredients in a small bowl.
2. Slice the ham into half inch pieces.
3. Spray the mixture with cooking spray.
4. Pre-heat the mixture over a medium-high heat.
5. Add the ham to the skillet and stir frequently for 3 to 5 minutes until the ham is warmed enough that it becomes crisped.
6. Remove it from the heat and keep aside.
7. Remove the yolk from boiled eggs and slice the remaining egg white and set it aside.
8. Toss the romaine and watercress in a large bowl with 2/3 of dressing.
9. Put the tomatoes on top by forming a row down in the middle.
10. Put the dressed greens on to the large serving dish.
11. Place the avocado, chicken, diced egg, crisped ham, and cheese in strips on either side of the tomatoes.
12. Sprinkle the remaining dressings and serve.

*Serves 6

ZESTY BLACK BEAN SALAD

Whether served as a salsa or eaten alone as a salad, this quick recipe is a great way to use up leftovers.

Ingredients:
1 cup black beans
¼ cup diced tomatoes
½ cup chopped bell peppers
Fresh cilantro
1 tsp. lime juice

Directions:
1. Mix the beans, tomatoes, bell peppers and lime juice in a bowl.
2. Finish by garnishing with fresh cilantro.

HAM AND CHEESE SALAD

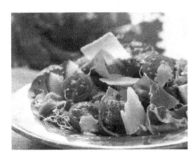

Ingredients:
2 cups romaine lettuce
4 ounces honey flavored ham
1 ounce part-skim mozzarella cheese, shredded
Cherry tomatoes sliced
½ cup sliced cucumber
2 tbsp. low-fat creamy Italian dressing

Directions:
1. Combine lettuce, tomatoes, cucumber, peppers, ham and mozzarella in a large bowl.
2. Mix in dressing and enjoy!

BOK CHOY SALAD WITH TURKEY BACON

Ingredients:
2 large carrots, thinly sliced
2 bunches baby bok choy, cut
6 ounces turkey bacon
1 can navy beans, drained and rinsed
1 cup grape or cherry tomatoes, halved
2 tbsp. fresh basil, chopped
2 tbsp. extra-virgin olive oil
2 tsp. lemon juice

Directions:
1. Steam carrots for four minutes. Then add bok choy stems and steam for one minute.
2. At the same time, cook bacon for one minute on each side. Slice when cool.
3. Mix all ingredients in a large bowl, add olive oil and lemon juice, toss, and serve.

SALAD GREENS, FETA AND GRAPES

Ingredients:
¼ cup extra-virgin olive oil
2 tbsp. red wine vinegar
¼ tsp. black ground pepper
8 cups salad greens of your choice
2 cups seedless grapes, halved
¾ cup feta cheese, crumbled

Directions:

1. Shake oil, vinegar, salt and pepper in a jar until blended.
2. Mix salad greens and lettuce in a large bowl.
3. Drizzle dressing on top and toss.
4. Add grapes and cheese and toss again.
5. Serve immediately.

*Serves 8

BLUE CHEESE AND APPLE SALAD

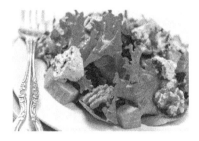

Ingredients:

1 cup romaine lettuce

1 small sliced apple

2 tbsp. pecans

1 tbsp. dried cranberries

2 tbsp. blue cheese crumbled

1 tbsp. olive oil

1 tbsp. apple cider vinegar

1 tsp. Dijon mustard

1 tsp. maple syrup

Directions:

1. Combine lettuce in a serving bowl and top with apple slices, pecans, cranberries, and blue cheese.
2. In a separate bowl, combine the oil, vinegar, mustard and syrup. Mix well and pour over salad.
3. Serve and enjoy!

SPICY ZUCCHINI NOODLE SALAD

Ingredients:
1 large zucchini squash
1 small bunch Italian kale
1 clove garlic, crushed
1 tbsp. fresh ginger, grated
1 tbsp. roasted sesame oil
1 tbsp. raw apple cider vinegar
1 tsp. roasted red chili flakes
Salt and pepper to taste

Directions:
1. Using a spiralizer, mandolin, or a large-slotted vegetable grater, slice zucchini into long noodle-like ribbons.
2. Transfer to a colander. Toss zucchini noodles with a pinch of salt and let drain for 30 minutes.
3. Slice Italian kale into thin ribbons and set aside.
4. In small bowl, whisk together garlic, ginger, roasted sesame oil, apple cider vinegar, and chili flakes until well combined.
5. In large bowl, add drained zucchini squash and Italian kale to. Slowly add dressing while simultaneously tossing with a pair of tongs to mix.
6. Serve immediately.

*Serves 2

ROAST BEEF SALAD

Ingredients:
3 ounces lean roast beef
½ cup red canned kidney beans, rinsed and drained
2 cups lettuce of your choice
½ cup chopped tomatoes
1 ounce low-fat shredded cheddar cheese
½ medium pear, sliced

1 tbsp. chopped walnuts

2 tbsp. reduced calorie Italian dressing

Directions:

1. Combine all of the above ingredients, toss and eat immediately.

SUMMER SALAD

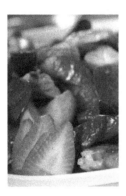

Ingredients:

Two cups of washed spinach leaves

1 chicken breast, cooked and chopped

1/2 cup strawberries, sliced

1/4 cup pecans, crumbled

1/2 cucumber, sliced

Directions:

1. In a bowl, combine all of the above ingredients.
2. Add sea salt and cracked black pepper to taste.
3. Serve with balsamic vinaigrette.

CHAPTER 7: 10 FUN SIDE DISHES & APPETIZERS

With several simple recipes on hand, eating clean will be no problem when it comes to preparing snacks. By keeping a variety of natural ingredients on hand that emphasizes the delicious flavors of fresh vegetables and herbs, one can always prepare a simple snack within a matter of minutes.

CARROT SOUP

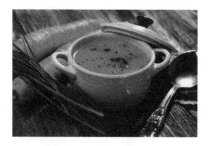

Ingredients:
2 tsp. dark sesame oil
½ cup plain Greek yogurt
1 tsp. grated ginger
1 lb. baby carrots, cut into 1 & 2 inch pieces
2 cups low sodium, fat- free chicken broth
1/3 cup sliced shallots
1 tbsp. olive oil

Directions:
1. Heat the olive oil in a medium sized saucepan, on medium high heat.
2. Add the shallots to the pan.

3. Cook shallots until almost tender, about 2 minutes, Stir Occasionally.
4. Add carrots and cook for 4 minutes
5. Add the chicken broth and bring to a boil.
6. Bring to low heat and simmer for 22 minutes until tender.
7. Add the grated ginger and cook for another 8 minutes, stirring occasionally.
8. Remove from heat covered and sit to cool for 5 minutes at room temperature.
9. Pour half the carrot mixture into a blender. Remove the center part of the blender lid to allow the steam to escape from blender. Put a towel over the open hole to avoid a mess.
10. Blend all ingredients until smooth.
11. Pour into a large bowl. Repeat this with the other half of the mixture.
12. Pour the blended ingredients back into the saucepan and heat on medium heat for about 2 minutes.
13. Pour into serving bowls and top with plain yogurt.

BAKED SWEET POTATO

Ingredients:
1 small sweet potato

Directions:
1. Puncture sweet potato with a fork and cook in microwave until done. (About 5 to 6 minutes.)
2. Peel if preferred and enjoy!

POTATOES WITH HERBS

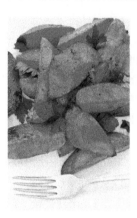

Ingredients:

1 pound new potatoes, halved

4 tsp. extra-virgin olive oil

2 tbsp. fresh parsley leaves, chopped

¼ tsp. kosher sea salt

1/8 tsp. black pepper

Directions:

1. Steam potatoes until tender, typically 10 to 15 minutes and place cooked potatoes in a large bowl, and add parsley, olive oil, salt, and pepper, and toss gently.
2. Serve while hot.

BAKED ONION RINGS

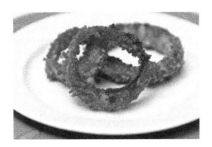

Ingredients:

1 large yellow onion sliced into desired thickness for rings

2 slices Ezekiel bread

1 egg

1 egg white

¼ cup oat flour

1/8 tsp. black pepper

1/8 tsp. garlic powder

A pinch of sea salt

Directions:

1. Preheat oven to 350 degrees.
2. Place bread on a baking sheet and toast until bread is hard but not burnt (8-10 minutes).
3. Let bread cool and then tear bread apart to make bread crumbs.
4. Combine egg and egg white in a bowl and whisk.
5. In another bowl combine bread crumbs, flour, black pepper, garlic powder and salt.
6. Dip each onion ring in egg mixture and then crumb mixture.
7. Place rings on a non-stick baking sheet.
8. Bake at 350 degrees for 8-10 minutes.

*Each onion should make about 20 rings if sliced into 1/3 inch rings.

EASY GUACAMOLE

Avocados are one of nature's wonder foods that can be used to prepare this fast snack that can be used as a spread or dip on whole-wheat pita chips.

Ingredients:
1 avocado
1 tbsp. minced garlic
1 tsp. lime juice
Sea salt to taste

Directions:
1. Mash one avocado in a bowl before adding minced garlic and lime juice.
2. Finish by adding a dash of sea salt and serve with warm pita chips or veggies.

STUFFED PEPPERS

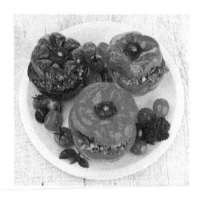

Ingredients:
4 bell peppers (with the tops sliced off and the stems and seeds removed)
1 cup lean minced beef
½ cup onions, chopped
½ cup chopped tomatoes
Pinch of sea salt

Pinch of cracked black pepper

1 tsp. garlic powder

Directions:

1. Preheat an oven to 370 degrees Fahrenheit.
2. Cook the minced beef until it is browned and then add the chopped onions.
3. Take the mixture off the flame once the onions have softened and become translucent.
4. Add the spices and tomatoes and mix thoroughly.
5. Put the peppers on a baking tray lined with foil.
6. Fill each of the peppers with the beef and onions and cook for 30 minutes.

RICOTTA STUFFED DATES

Ingredients:

¼ cup light ricotta cheese

¼ tbsp. ground cardamom

1 tbsp. honey (raw)

2 tbsp. ground pistachios (raw)

12 blanched almonds (raw)

12 medium deglet nour dates

Directions:

1. Stir ricotta and honey together in a small bowl.
2. Then add the ground pistachios and cardamom.
3. Then slice each date lengthwise with a knife and stuff the dates with about a tbsp. of the ricotta mix.
4. Add a single pistachio to the top of the date as a garnish.

TZATZIKI SAUCE

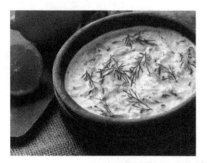

This traditional Greek sauce is often served alongside gyros, but here it provides the perfect dip in include on a veggie tray.

Ingredients:
2 cups Greek yogurt
2 tbsp. lemon juice
1 minced garlic clove
1 large cucumber, diced
1 tsp. salt
1 tsp. each of fresh dill and mint

Directions:
1. Except for the yogurt, place all ingredients into a food processor and process until it is well-blended.
2. Then, stir the mixture into the Greek yogurt.
3. Sea salt and black pepper can be added to taste.

Although this recipe is best when it is allowed to sit in the refrigerator, it is still delicious when eaten right away. Simply serve alongside a tray of fresh vegetables and encourage everyone to use it as a dip.

SLICED TOMATOES & FETA

Ingredients:
2 large ripe tomatoes, sliced (8 slices)

2 tbsp. low-fat crumbled feta cheese

1 tbsp. balsamic vinegar

2 tbsp. fresh minced basil

Ground pepper to taste

Directions:
1. Slice tomatoes and arrange on a plate.
2. Sprinkle with feta cheese.
3. Drizzle tomatoes with vinegar.
4. Sprinkle with basil and pepper.

*4 servings

SWEET POTATO FRIES

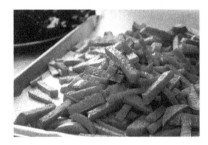

Ingredients:
1 pound sweet potatoes

1 tbsp. olive oil

¼ tsp. kosher sea salt

1 tsp. fresh rosemary, chopped

Directions:
1. Preheat oven to 425 degrees Fahrenheit.
2. Combine olive oil and rosemary in a small bowl.
3. Clean and slice potatoes into wedges or slices.
4. Toss potatoes with olive oil-rosemary mixture.
5. Spread potatoes on a parchment-lined baking sheet. Bake for 35 minutes, flipping potatoes halfway through the baking time.
6. Remove from oven, sprinkle with salt, and serve.

CHAPTER 8: 10 WHOLESOME CLEAN EATING DINNER RECIPES

At the end of a long day, it can be difficult to find the energy to cook a healthy and delicious meal. Here are ten ideas for dinner that taste great, are good for you, and are easy to make.

GARLIC-RUBBED CHICKEN BREAST WITH STEAMED ASPARAGUS AND LEMON DILL GREEK YOGURT DIPPING SAUCE

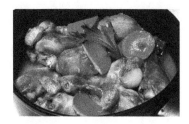

Ingredients:
2 chicken breasts
2 cloves of garlic, peeled and with one end chopped off
1 bundle of asparagus
Sea salt and cracked black pepper to taste
1 cup of Greek-style yoghurt
1 tbsp. of lemon juice
¼ cup of fresh dill

Directions:
1. Add a tbsp. of oil to a pan and cook the chicken breasts until a knife test shows they are no longer pink in the middle.
2. Rub the chicken breasts with the garlic cloves and add salt and pepper to taste.
3. Trim the ends of the asparagus and steam until they are fork tender, but not soft.

4. In a bowl, combine the Greek-style yoghurt, lemon juice, and dill.
5. Serve as a dipping sauce for the asparagus or the chicken, whichever is preferred.

CHICKEN BREAST STUFFED WITH AVOCADO AND RED ONION

Ingredients:
2 chicken breasts (cook and butterfly)

1 avocado, mashed

¼ cup chopped red onion

Sea salt and cracked black pepper to taste

Directions:
1. In a bowl, combine the avocado, red onion, sea salt, and cracked black pepper.
2. Spoon into the center of the butterfly chicken breasts and close them.
3. Serve with a green salad.

QUICK LAMB STEW WITH BELL PEPPERS, ONIONS, AND CARROTS

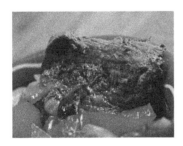

Ingredients:
1 pound of diced lamb

2 bell peppers, diced

½ cup of chopped onions

1 carrot, peeled and chopped

2 cloves of garlic, peeled and crushed

2 cans of chopped tomatoes

1 tsp. of chili powder

Sea salt and cracked black pepper to taste

Directions:

1. Add two tbsp. of oil to a deep pan and place it on medium heat.
2. Add the diced lamb and cook until the meat is no longer pink. Add the bell peppers, onions, and carrots, and cook until they are soft.
3. Stir in the garlic, chili powder, and the salt and pepper. Add the chopped tomatoes, and turn the heat down to low.
4. Cover the pan and let the stew cook for another fifteen minutes.

This dish will keep well and tastes even better the next day.

ALMOND CRUSTED SHRIMP

Ingredients:

½ cup ground almonds

1 tsp. parsley

3 tbsp. all-purpose flour

½ tsp. seafood seasoning

¼ tsp. sea salt

¼ tsp. black pepper

1 lb. shrimp, peeled and deveined

2 tsp. almond oil

1 lemon cut into wedges

2 tbsp. almond oil

Directions:

1. Stir together almonds, flour, parsley, seafood seasoning, salt and pepper.
2. Dip each shrimp in egg white and then in almond mixture.
3. Lay on a baking sheet or platter until ready to cook.

4. Heat 1 tbsp. oil in a large skillet and grill shrimp on medium heat, cooking 3 to 4 minutes until pink and golden.
5. Serve shrimp accompanied by lemon wedges.

PORK LOIN CUTLET WITH SAUTEED MUSHROOM, ONIONS AND BROCCOLI

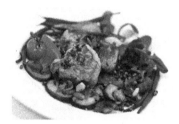

Ingredients:
2 pork loin cutlets
1 cup mushrooms, washed and chopped
½ cup onions, diced
1 cup broccoli
1 garlic clove, crushed

Directions:
1. In a pan, cook the pork loin cutlets until they are no longer pink.
2. Add salt and pepper to taste and set aside.
3. Add a tbsp. of oil and sauté the mushrooms, onions, and garlic.
4. Once these are cooked, pour the mixture over the pork loins.
5. Steam the broccoli, add salt and pepper to taste, and serve.

CHICKEN AND APRICOT TAGINE

Ingredients:
4 chicken breasts, chopped
1 cup of dried apricots
½ cup chopped onions
1 tsp. of chili powder
Pinch of cinnamon

2 cloves of garlic, crushed

Sea salt and cracked black pepper to taste

2 cans of chopped tomatoes

Directions:

1. Add a tbsp. of oil to a pan and cook the chicken breasts on medium heat until they are no longer pink.
2. Add the onions.
3. When the onions have softened, add the apricots, chili powder, cinnamon, garlic, salt, and pepper. Stir in the chopped tomatoes.
4. Transfer the mixture to a casserole dish and place in the oven at 180 degrees Fahrenheit for 25 minutes.
5. This is even tastier the following day.

STUFFED TURKEY BURGERS

Ingredients:

1 lb. lean ground turkey

2 tomatoes

1 cup shredded mozzarella cheese

2 tbsp. balsamic vinegar

2 tbsp. basil leaves

1 tbsp. onion powder

1 tsp. garlic powder

1 tsp. Italian seasoning

Directions:

1. Season the ground turkey with the garlic powder, Italian seasoning and onion powder.
2. Separate the ground turkey into 4 equal portions.
3. Roll the turkey portions into balls and flatten out. Make a dent in the middle of the patties.
4. In the middle of your patty sprinkle ¼ cup of mozzarella. Next add the sliced tomatoes and basil. Top with another ¼ cup of mozzarella.

5. Place a plain patty on top of the prepared patty.
6. Pinch the edges of the two patties together in an attempt to seal them.
7. Cook on medium heat in a covered frying pan for 15 minutes or until thoroughly cooked. Can also be grilled.

*Serves 2

CRAB CAKES

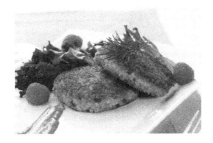

Ingredients:
1½ cups bread crumbs
¼ cup green onions, chopped
2 tbsp. fresh dill, chopped
2 tbsp. reduced fat mayonnaise
¼ tsp. black pepper
2 egg whites
1 lb. crab meat (no shell)
1 tbsp. canola oil
Cooking spray

Directions:
1. Combine bread crumbs, onions, dill, mayonnaise, pepper, egg whites and crab meat.
2. Divide this mixture into 6 equal portions, making 1-inch-thick patties.
3. Heat oil in a large skillet over medium-high heat.
4. Cook patties 1 minute on each side.

5. Finish up by baking the patties at a pre-heated 400 degrees for 20 minutes.

*Serves 6

VEGETABLE QUESADILLAS

Ingredients:
Whole wheat tortilla
Low fat shredded cheese
Black beans, canned
Shredded carrot, broccoli or cabbage
Salsa

Directions:
1. Warm tortilla in a heated pan.
2. Add cheese.
3. Add black beans, rinsed and drained.
4. Add slaw of your choice
5. Add more cheese and another tortilla.
6. Cook until cheese is melted and tortillas are golden brown.
7. Slice into wedges and serve with salsa.

RED WINE PORK CHOPS

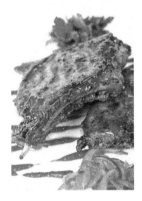

Ingredients:

2 cups dry red wine

5 bay leaves

2 tbsp. fresh, minced rosemary

1½ tsp. ground coriander

½ tsp. ground cloves

½ tsp. ground nutmeg

6 1½-inch thick boneless loin chips

Sea salt and cracked black pepper to taste

Directions:

1. Combine red wine, bay leaves, rosemary, coriander, nutmeg, and cloves in a glass dish.
2. Place chops in marinade mixture.
3. Marinate overnight in refrigerator, turning occasionally.
4. Drain chops and pat dry; discard used marinade.
5. Season with salt and pepper and lightly brush with olive oil.
6. Grill the chops over medium high heat for 6 to 8 minutes on each side.
7. Serve and enjoy!

*Serves 6

CHAPTER 9: 10 YUMMY CLEAN EATING DESSERT RECIPES

The diet of clean eating is one in which an eater attempts to consume foods in their most natural and whole state. This means foods like vegetables and fruits as well as foods that feature healthy fats instead of saturated fat. One of the interesting facets of this diet is that it's not one where the most important factor is counting calories. Dieters instead focus on ensuring each food they eat is as healthy as possible.

The following delicious desserts are a wonderful way to end a day of healthy and nutritious clean eating.

WATERMELON SMOOTHIE

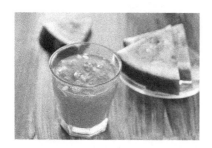

Ingredients:
3 cups watermelon, seedless and cubed
1 tbsp. sugar
2 tbsp. lime juice
1 cup crushed ice
½ cup water

Directions:
1. Combine all the above ingredients in a blender until smooth.

NATURAL BROWNIES

Ingredients:

1½ tbsp. raw cocoa powder

2 tbsp. natural granola

3 drops dark chocolate Stevia

¼ cup cottage cheese

3 egg whites

Directions:

1. Pre-heat the oven to 350 degrees.
2. Mix cocoa powder, cottage cheese, egg whites, and sweetener (use a blender to mix ingredients exceptionally well).
3. Pour the mixture into a square brownie baking tin.
4. Bake for about 5 minutes and take the tin out of the oven.
5. Sprinkle the granola over the top of the brownies.
6. Bake for another 15 minutes.

CHEESECAKE

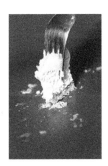

Ingredients:

¼ cup plain yogurt

1/3 cup unrefined sugar cane

1/3 cup evaporated cane juice

2 tbsp. water

2 eggs (large)

6 ounces cream cheese (light)

Directions:

1. Preheat oven to 350 degrees Fahrenheit.
2. While the oven heats up, combine the unrefined sugar cane with 2 tbsp. of water and bring the mixture to a boil.
3. Stir the mixture for a short time after the boiling point and then pour the mixture into a set of 6 small ramekins.
4. Then mix the cane juice, cream cheese, eggs, and yogurt in a separate bowl until the mixture is sufficiently combined.
5. Pour the new mixture into the ramekins.
6. Take a large baking pan and fill it halfway with warm water.
7. Place each of the ramekins in the pan (as if they were swimming) and bake for about a half hour.

EASY BANANA NUT COOKIES

Having these banana nut cookies on hand will always be a great way to provide a fast snack. A healthier alternative to sugary store bought cookies; this recipe only requires three natural ingredients.

Ingredients:
2 overripe bananas
1 cup steel-cut oats
½ cup chopped pecans

Directions:
1. Mash the overripe bananas by hand until they are completely softened.
2. Then, mix in the oats and pecans.
3. Use a spoon to place mounds on a cookie sheet before placing them in an oven pre-heated to 350 degrees for 15 minutes.

BROWN RICE PUDDING

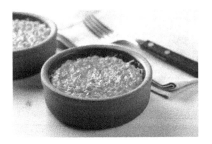

Ingredients:

1 tsp. unrefined sugar cane

1/8 tsp. nutmeg

½ tsp. vanilla extract

1/8 tbsp. nutmeg

1 tbsp. blackstrap molasses

½ cup low-fat milk

1 cup cooked long-grain brown rice

6 egg whites

Directions:

1. Boil rice and milk on the stovetop.
2. Add egg whites to mixture, stirring constantly until the egg whites are cooked.
3. Add the rest of the ingredients by stirring them into the mixture.

ORANGE DELIGHT

Ingredients:

40 almonds

4 oranges, peeled

1½ cups low-fat plain yogurt

Directions:

1. Mix almonds, yogurt, and oranges and enjoy as dessert.

BAKED APPLE SURPRISE

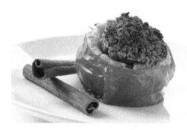

Ingredients:
1 large apple, cored and halved

2 tsp. reduced fat cream cheese

1 small pear, cored and cubed

½ tsp. organic brown sugar

1/8 tsp. ground cinnamon

2 tsp. cinnamon

1 tbsp. chopped almonds

3 tbsp. water or apple juice

Directions:
1. Preheat oven to 350 degrees Fahrenheit.
2. Slice apple in half.
3. Scoop out some apple flesh from each half leaving room for filling. Add cream cheese in the cavity of each half.
4. Dice pear. Toss pear with brown sugar and cinnamon.
5. Fill each apple half with diced pear.
6. Sprinkle pear filling with almonds.
7. Place apple halves in a baking dish and add water or apple juice.
8. Cover and bake for 30 minutes, then baste with juices and bake uncovered for 10 minutes or until almonds are roasted.

CARROT BREAD

Ingredients:
½ tsp. nutmeg

½ tsp. vanilla extract

¼ tsp. salt

1½ tsp.baking soda

2 tsp. cinnamon

2 tbsp. olive oil

2 tbsp. natural apple juice

¼ cup raisins

¾ cup agave nectar

¾ cup water

1½ cup whole wheat flour

1½ cup carrots (shredded)

1 egg white

1 egg

Directions:
1. Mix together flour, carrots, raisins, cinnamon, salt, baking soda, nutmeg, and 1/2 cup agave nectar.
2. In the middle of this mixture, pour the oil, water, and eggs into the bowl.
3. Stir everything together until it is nicely combined.
4. Pour mixture into pan and bake for about 45 minutes.
5. During the baking, combine the remaining agave nectar, vanilla extract, and apple juice for the glaze.
6. When the bread comes out of the oven, drape the glaze over the finished bread.

CHOCOLATE COVERED BANANA BITES

Ingredients:
2 ripe bananas

½ cup dark chocolate chips

2 tbsp. unsweetened coconut

Directions:

1. Peel ripe bananas.
2. Cut up into 1-2 inch bites.
3. Put chocolate chips into a microwave for 30-45 seconds in a microwave safe dish.
4. Stir well until chips are melted and the chocolate is a smooth consistency.
5. Place banana bites into chocolate and roll around to coat. (Use toothpicks)
6. Place chocolate covered banana chunks on a piece of wax paper.
7. Sprinkle with coconut flakes. (Optional)
8. Place the banana chunks in the freezer to harden.
9. Serve and enjoy

OATMEAL RAISIN COOKIES WITH CINNAMON

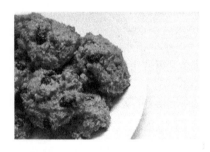

Ingredients:

¼ cup sea salt

½ cup natural applesauce

½ cup raisins

½ tsp. of baking powder

1/3 cup unrefined sugar cane

1 tsp. cinnamon

1 tsp. pure vanilla extract

2 tbsp. water

2 egg whites

2/3 cup pastry flour (whole wheat)

2 cup oats

Directions:

1. Preheat oven to 350 degrees Fahrenheit.
2. Mix all the ingredients together in a bowl and spoon mixture onto a non-stick baking sheet in small, cookie-sized balls.
3. Flatten the balls with the palm of your hand before baking.
4. Bake for about 15 minutes.

With the right recipes, clean eating can be the way to a healthier number on the scale and may also be the best way to enjoy a long and disease-free life. Many dieters are so used to eating high amounts of saturated fat and added sugars that switching to clean eating may be difficult. Creativity with recipe choice will ensure anyone can stick with this diet and lead a healthier lifestyle.

ABOUT THE AUTHOR

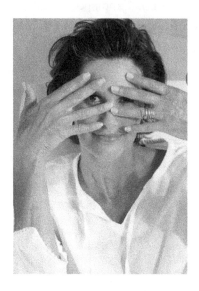

Author and chef Daisy Williams is passionate about clean and healthy eating, but she knows that it can seem next to impossible to someone just embarking on a food journey. It took years for her to move from the all-American diet processed and chemical-ridden convenience food to a healthier lifestyle that draws true nourishment from organic, whole foods. Now that she's made the transition herself, she loves helping people realize that there is a healthier way and that it's not as hard as you might think!

Eating clean didn't come easily to Daisy—her food journey started out of pure necessity. After being constantly ill for years and trying just about every medicine under the sun, she finally tried the nutrition angle as a last-ditch effort. A friend had advised reducing the chemicals in her diet, and since nothing else seemed to be working, she figured there was nothing to lose. Within weeks it became clear that nutrition was a huge factor impacting her health concerns! And thus her passion for clean eating was born.

Daisy is convinced that most people can improve their quality of life by adjusting their nutritional lifestyle. And she wants people considering clean eating to know that it's not impossible; in fact, it's delicious! Her books feature some fantastic recipes, from clean eating, green smoothies to Paleo slow cooker recipes that you'll love. Her dream is that through her story, people will be inspired to make healthy changes even before their health is suffering.

MORE BOOKS BY DAISY WILLIAMS

Clean Eating: Your Guide For Eating Clean

Green Smoothies: The 50 Best Green Smoothie Recipes For Weight Loss – How to Make the Best Green Smoothies to Drop Pounds

Paleo Slow Cooker Recipes: The Best Paleo Diet Recipes For Your Slow Cooker

CPSIA information can be obtained
at www.ICGtesting.com
Printed in the USA
LVHW061354290319
612328LV00005B/44/P